SURVIVAL OF THE FIT

How I Listened to
My Doctor & Lost 100 Pounds

Michael Alan Grapin

Cover design & typography by Stephen D. Sullivan.

For Dr. Agarwal.

Chapter One

Some people can eat anything they want and never gain weight; I'm not one of those people. I've struggled with my weight for my entire life and I believe it has to do as much with my mind set as anything else. I needed to escape the repeated cycle of losing and regaining substantial amounts of excess weight.

Like most dieters, I've lost and gained my total body weight several times over during the course of my lifetime. I come from a family in which we all had issues with our weight and dealt with it in different manners. One fad diet or another usually led to temporary weight loss and preening, but a return to normal eating resulted in a rebounding weight gain each and every time for all but one of my sisters who did whatever she could to remain svelte and the belle of the ball.

There were psychological issues that haunt me to this day. I've never been able to get past being told I must clean my plate because there are children starving in one part of the world or another. Wasting food was a great sin in my family of overeating foodies. Another sin was failing to have enough food for everyone who came to the table. We seemed to require enough food to fill our plates several times and still maintain room for dessert. And yet, to this very day, leftovers can make the cook pout.

I'm writing this on recommendation of one of my doctors who believes my achievement nothing short of extraordinary. Many people have asked me how I did it. Well everyone, this is how I did it. I can't guarantee that this will work for you, but I can assure you that it worked for me. If you find inspiration in my success that leads to your own success story, so be it!

As I begin to write this, I weigh below 169 pounds. Less than a year ago I was admitted to the hospital with chest pains and had to undergo a couple of angioplasties to clear my clogged arteries. When I was first admitted, the nursing staff weighed me in at 260 pounds. My visit to the emergency room may have been the impetus to make my lifestyle change, but it took more than that for me to stick with it and lose over 90 pounds in a year.

Before I continue, I feel a little background is in order. That particular trip to the hospital was not my first and we need to go back about fifteen years to begin my story. I was forty-two and 250 pounds, we were dining out with another couple when I felt the first chest pain that really shook me. I had been living with mild chest pains for years at that point and always attributed them to over exertion. I assumed that it was my body's way of telling me that I'd over done it and it was time for a rest. This was different. I was seated in a restaurant in a relaxed atmosphere as I felt short of breath and pain radiated from the center of my chest up to my jaw and down my arm.

At that time, I couldn't recall the last time I'd seen a doctor. Hey, I'm a guy and it is common knowledge amongst the women I know that we guys are notorious about being lax in taking care of ourselves. My wife and I asked around for a recommendation which led to my first visit with Dr. Radel. I described my reason for seeing him and was told my symptoms were classic. He immediately prescribed a beta blocker, Lipitor and baby aspirin. I was given Nitroglycerin and instructed how to use it – I was to place one under my tongue when angina flared, sit down and rest. If the pain hadn't subsided within a half hour, I was to take another pill and call an ambulance. He also made an appointment for me with a cardiologist for an angiogram bypassing a stress test that he didn't believe I would survive.

Back then, an angiogram that indicated an angioplasty was required would mean two separate procedures about a week apart. At least that was the preferred scenario. My angiogram which indicated a 99% blockage also resulted in a small tear in my femoral artery as the catheter was removed. Because my insurance company limited the length of time I was permitted to stay in the hospital, I was released and sent home to await my angioplasty to be performed the following week. What hadn't been planned was the internal bleeding that resulted from the tear which quickly led to a subdural hematoma that required an emergency return to the hospital and surgery to repair the tear. Naturally the cardiologist assured me that this was a freak occurrence and apologized profusely so I stuck with him for the angioplasty that was scheduled a week after I was sent home following my second release from the hospital. In retrospect, this was not the best decision I could have made. Complications arose from the angioplasty that landed me in the cardiac care unit until my vitals stabilized, but they still found it best to send me home as soon as possible because of my health care coverage.

So to say I found the whole experience off-putting is really putting it mildly. My trust for the whole medical community in general was reduced, but I still had faith in Dr. Radel. I liked his bedside manner and sense of humor – I remember one time, while he was administering a prostate exam, I made some glib remark about how much I was enjoying the procedure and he replied, "Good, next time I'll use my finger." -- I decided that I would follow his advice and hope for the best. He suggested something that he called "The Sensible Diet" that required the elimination of all wheat products from my diet. There was a list of acceptable fruits and vegetables, proteins and starches. I came to think of it as the chicken and broccoli diet, since that was mostly what I ate for dinner. I avoided bread, rice and pasta. I could have a dry baked potato, or some roasted potatoes, but nothing in the way of French fries, scalloped potatoes, mashed potatoes or potatoes au gratin. Breakfast was a bowl of oatmeal, a snack was celery and if I felt hungry I could fill up on a green salad or a glass of diet soda such as Fresca.

I stuck to this diet and lost weight rapidly. Six months later, Dr. Radel allowed me to join a gym and work out with a trainer twice a week although he wasn't thrilled with me lifting weights. My weight got down below 180 pounds, I looked and felt great. I became convinced that I was in the best shape of my life and decided to join a softball league. I had been pretty good at softball when I was a kid, but as an adult who hadn't played the game in more than twenty years I was considerably less than great. I couldn't hit worth a damn and my throwing was inaccurate at best, but at least I was a slow runner. Actually I think it safe to say that I was the worst player in the league, but I stuck with it and played badly for two full seasons. Eventually I took pity on my team mates and hung up my cleats.

Through it all I worked with Dr. Radel to improve my health one issue at a time. My diet was a constant source of concern and I kept getting conflicting signals. I was told to fill up on vegetables if I wanted to snack, but during one examination Dr. Radel noticed discoloring of my skin which indicated that I was eating far too many vegetables and should lay off the carrots in particular. At one point, the good doctor told me that a glass of red wine offered benefits to a heart patient because of the anti oxidants called flavonoids, but later decided that my rise in triglycerides could be attributed to the wine and told me to cut it out. There was a point at which I was diagnosed with bipolar disorder and given lithium and tranquilizers to stabilize my mood swings. I hated taking the meds because of the way they made me feel, so we explored diet once again. We tried eliminating sugar, caffeine and alcohol finding that my moods stabilized. One by one, each was returned to my diet until it was determined that I was sensitive to caffeine. I was delighted to learn that if I drank decaffeinated tea I could have sugar and alcohol in moderation.

Then the problems began. My weight had been under control for years following my heart problems, but my nature once again reared its ugly head. At one point I was able to get Dr. Radel to admit that wheat wasn't actually a health issue and that I had only been told to eliminate it from my diet in order to help me lose weight. It was suggested that I could begin to eat bread and pasta in moderation. Of course the problem was that I couldn't do anything in moderation. I've always been an obsessive eater. I didn't want a slice of bread, I wanted the whole loaf! I couldn't stop at one slice of pizza, I wanted the whole pie. One scoop of ice-cream wasn't enough, I craved the whole quart! And to make matters worse, I thought I could handle eating more because of my regular visits to the gym. Then I tried to convince myself that my gradual weight gain was due to increased muscle mass because everyone knew that muscle weighs more than fat.

I was only kidding myself and losing control. I got lazy and began looking for excuses not to exercise. A brief financial down turn convinced me that I couldn't afford to maintain the cost of my expensive gym. I further convinced myself that I could exercise at home with what I'd learned from my personal trainer; which might have been true if I had stuck with it. Bit by bit, I reverted to old eating habits. As my weight increased, I actually became embarrassed to see my doctor convinced he would scold me for my bad behavior.

My prescriptions ran out and Dr. Radel insisted that I had to come to see him before he would renew them. I felt fine, so I said the hell with it and stopped taking the prescribed medication…I wasn't going to be held hostage by prescriptions! I convinced myself that I could get by with aspirin, fish oil and Centrum Cardio. Soon after that Dr. Radel retired and I hit my fiftieth birthday. I even told myself that no one cares if some guy over fifty gets fat and just let myself eat anything I wanted. Disaster!

I was my own worst enemy. My return to obesity was a slow process. My wife packed away successively larger jeans as I outgrew them. My waist eventually swelled to over forty-eight inches and I had jeans measuring every two inches from thirty-four inches on up.

I've had a beard continuously since I was a teenager. As I got heavier, I let my beard grown longer and fuller thinking that it better suited my thickening physique. My beard that had once been auburn was now showing increasing amounts of grey. The graying made for interesting reactions from those who saw me. The longer and grayer my beard got, the nicer people seemed to act toward me. I began encountering small children who would shyly ask if I was Santa Claus and I would play along telling them that I was. I'd claim that whatever they saw me doing was what I did in the off season and being there was how I kept my eye on them to learn if they were naughty or nice.

Along the way, I acquired a Santa suit from a costume shop nearby where I live. I played Santa in a parade or two, waving to the crowd from behind the wheel of my red Smart Car. I posed for a photographer with an interesting sense of humor who had me dressed up as Santa with an orthodox Jewish child sitting on my lap and used our image on his holiday cards. I was frequently told that I would make a wonderful Santa. At one point I considered accepting a gig as a department store Santa and looked into what that might entail. I loved the adoration and it even inspired me to write a novel in which there is an army of Santas who act as the front men for the elves who actually run the entire operation (check out my novel, *Santa 17*).

Obviously I was being an idiot. The chest pains had returned, but I chose to ignore them and tried to convince myself that they were due to over exertion once again. I didn't have a doctor to consult with and I was disenchanted with the whole medical profession because of my experiences of fourteen years before. It was becoming increasingly apparent that something was wrong. I couldn't make it up a flight of stairs without gasping for air. As long as I could make the chest pains subside with a bit of rest and a belch, I could fool myself into believe everything would be fine. I was living on Pepcid Complete for my acid reflux and heartburn; and I frequently had to sleep sitting up. Looking back, I have to believe that my excessive weight was contributing to my sciatica and arthritis. There were times I needed a cane to walk and I often had trouble holding a pencil because my hand was swollen and ached so badly. I knew my blood pressure was through the roof and had been told on more than one occasion that I was a stroke waiting to happen. I told myself that I wasn't afraid to die and would go to bed some nights hoping that I wouldn't awaken in the morning.

Then one evening the chest pains wouldn't subside. My wife saw the stricken expression upon my face and asked if I was alright. I admitted that I was having chest pains. She asked if I wanted to go to the emergency room. I insisted that I didn't want to go but thought that I probably should; ever the wise guy, yes indeed, that's me!

It's interesting to note that when you enter the emergency room at Valley Hospital in Ridgewood, New Jersey and complain of chest pains, you get moved to the front of the line. In no time they determined that my blood pressure was way too high. I think it was something like 210/105. They gave me Nitroglycerin and brought me to the Cardiac care unit where they set about stabilizing my vital signs in preparation for a procedure performed by a cardiologist.

The cardiologist informed me that I had something he called a cardiac episode and he was going to perform an angiogram, but unlike fourteen years before, if a blockage was found an angioplasty would be performed immediately. A lot of changes had been made to the whole procedure I'd undergone fourteen years before many of which appeared designed to prevent the very complications I'd experienced the time before. Several blockages were found requiring three different angioplasties and seven new stents all told over a number of months.

Although the cardiologist wouldn't call what I had a heart attack, the nurses assured me that, of course, I did have a heart attack and that I was an idiot for going off my meds and ignoring the warning signs for so long. Because I didn't want to continue taking two prescription medications I now needed to take seven including something for type two diabetes. To make matters all the more confusing, I had two doctors to deal with in the hospital both named Dr. Agarwal who were, oddly enough, unrelated to one another.

Dr. Agarwal, the cardiologist, wanted assurances that I would behave before he went ahead and performed the procedures. Dr. Agarwal, the internist, prescribed the medications and coordinated meetings with a diabetes consultant and a dietician. Dr. Agarwal, the internist, and the dietician laid out what they called a workable diet advising that I needed to cut out desserts, cut back on my portions, avoid white flour and white rice and white potatoes. I should stick to whole grains, brown rice and yams. Grilled, baked or roasted fish, chicken, turkey and pork were fine, beef no more than once a week, lots of vegetables and fresh fruit, so on and so forth. Dr. Agarwal, the internist, advised moderate exercise, but no heavy lifting for a while, and assured me that it is always his aim to get his patients off of the medications down the road. If I lost as little as twenty pounds, I might be able to get off of the diabetes medication.

Talk about your classic carrot and stick. He listened carefully to my story about the complications that arose those fourteen years before and claimed he understood my distrust of the medical profession based on that experience. He listened to my feelings about taking medication and being held hostage by my prescriptions. I would later learn that he didn't expect me to actually follow his recommendations. He gives everyone the same sort of advice and has come to learn that he is usually ignored.

I'm not sure what it was that resonated with me, but I was fifty-six years old and weighed 260 pounds; I listened to what everyone had to say and decided to pay attention. I distilled all of the advice that I was given while in the hospital down into a manageable course of action.

Michael Alan Grapin

I'm not going to claim that what I did and what I'm continuing to do now will work for everyone. I really have no idea if it will or won't work for you. However, I can say without fear of contradiction that it worked for me. So what follows is how I did it and if you can somehow adapt it for yourself and make it work for you as well, I think that would be fantastic!

Chapter Two

As I suggested at the beginning, I've often succeeded at diets in the past only to put all the weight and more back on over time after the diet allowed me to reach my goal and I resumed eating "normally". I've come to think that the biggest problem with the diet mentality is thinking of it as an abnormal or unnatural way of eating. Obviously, being on a diet was never a guarantee of success in the long term for me. I'm hoping that I don't repeat past mistakes, but I suspect that the problem for me has always been one of perception. If I think of the diet as temporary, I'm doomed to repeat the cycle.

Therefore, I'm not on a diet this time; instead I've made a lifestyle change. I've changed my eating habits permanently. I have to understand that this will be the way I eat for the rest of my life; I cannot resume previous eating habits. It's a mindset just as accepting that leftovers are good and that it is better to waste food than have it add to my waist. I simply needed to find new eating habits that I could live with forever; how difficult could that possibly be, right?

I've had to adapt my new eating habits through trial and error. Being prescribed Atorvastatin, Pantaprazole, Metoprolol tartr, Amlodipine Besylate, Effient, Diovan and Januvia had an immediate influence on my evolving eating habits. As I mentioned before, Dr. Agarwal, the internist, was aware of my aversion toward taking prescription medication and dangled a carrot; he would reduce the number/dosages of medications if I managed to lose sufficient weight. However, the weight loss in and of itself was secondary to learning to eat a healthy diet.

Januvia was to dictate my new eating habits the most profoundly since it forced me to eat on a schedule; I couldn't skip meals because my blood sugar would drop and I would get light headed. I had to eat breakfast and be prepared with a snack for mid morning just in case I began feeling dizzy. Consultants in the hospital had explained about ratios of carbohydrates to soluble fiber which had my wife and me reading nutrition labels as never before.

Fellow diabetics offered tips and advice about the mid-morning snack that varied from a Lifesaver candy, to grapes, to snack bars approved by the Diabetes Association. It was interesting to note that once it was known that I had been diagnosed as type two diabetic I was immediately welcomed into a large community of fellow sufferers eager to offer advice on everything from snacks, to meals and sugar substitutes. I had been unaware about the plight of dear friends and relatives with the disease. A salesman I'd known for years and my wife's coworker were among my new advisors. All had something to contribute to my growing knowledge about living with diabetes, but once again it was up to me to distill all of that advice and turn it into something that would work for me.

We were given a device to test my blood sugar levels and instructed in its use. It was to become a valuable gauge of what I could and couldn't eat. Contrary to what I had been instructed by the diabetes expert in the hospital, Dr. Agarwal, the internist, suggested that we needed to test my blood sugar level no more than once a day about two hours after eating. My wife and I got into the habit of testing my sugar in the evening after my last meal of the day. As long as my level was below 150, what I had eaten was acceptable. If something I ate caused my sugar level to rise over the 150 mark, in the future I should avoid eating whatever it was that I had eaten to cause the elevated levels. I was surprised to learn, for example, that Chinese food caused my sugar to spike; I'd always considered it one of the healthier cuisines. A little research indicated that much Chinese cuisine is very high in sugar. I've actually learned to enjoy the steamed chicken and vegetables (without any sauce) and brown rice offered by most Chinese restaurants. It was either that or I would have to begin to avoid places like "The Hunan Gourmet" altogether which certainly wouldn't be fair to my wife who craves her fix of General Tso's Chicken now and then.

Reducing sugar in my diet was as easy as eliminating most desserts and drinking nothing but water. I was genuinely surprised at how much sugar and calories were to be found in every sort of fruit juice. I'd believed that orange juice, grapefruit juice or Ocean Spray blueberry/cranberry juice cocktail made a preferable and healthy substitute for soda and other soft drinks. At least fruit juices were full of nutrients and anti-oxidants, not the empty calories to be found in soda or Country Time lemonade, right? I couldn't have been more wrong, apparently. A recent study suggests that the fructose in fruit juice is quite fattening without the dietary fiber to counteract it. As soon as I began drinking nothing but water and the occasional cup of decaf tea sweetened with Equal, the weight began to come off.

Equal was my artificial sweetener of choice. I've tried the pink and yellow packets as well, but the little blue packets were the most palatable to me. If artificial sweeteners are to be a part of your future, I think you'll have to try them all until you find the one that appeals most to you. I did find all sorts of negative press about aspartame which increased my levels of stress for a period, but after a long conversation with a dietician who is seeing one of my cousins, I was assured that the quantities I was consuming were of little or no danger to me.

The decision to drink nothing but water also meant that I had to change my pre-meal habit in a restaurant. When asked if I want anything to drink before dinner now, I eschew that glass of Merlot, I forego that Pina Colada and no longer indulge in that tasty pitcher of sangria at Jalapeño's.

I haven't had any cake, pie, cookies, pudding or ice-cream in about a year. Although the diabetic snack bars resembled a candy bar, I haven't had any real chocolate from Hannah Krause's Home Made Candies, Hershey's or Nestles in more than a year; and I don't miss it! Now and forever more, dessert will be fresh fruit or a small container of Dannon light & fit yogurt, I'm particularly fond of the peach, blueberry and strawberry flavors and it's an added bonus that they now indicate they are free of aspartame – why take chances, right? My wife and I have even gotten into the habit of referring to my containers of yogurt as pudding – we're just too cute at times. Substituting fruit for other desserts is no hardship for me as I really like fresh fruit, but I've had to make adjustments with that as well. Even fruit should be enjoyed in moderation.

My other issues with fruit, however, include how perishable most can be. I still harbor residual problems with allowing food to go bad. Care must be taken in how much quantity we purchase so I won't be tempted to eat too much rather than allowing it to spoil. I've found that certain fruits keep better than others and offer a wider window of opportunity for consumption. For example, I find that bananas are optimal to be eaten for only a couple of days, whereas apples and oranges will keep in the refrigerator for weeks.

My innate laziness is also a contributing factor in my fruit choices. A lot of fruit requires varying degrees of preparation and I find myself choosing the path of least resistance. Grapes or berries are ready to eat after rinsing. However, peeling an orange is just more effort than sectioning an apple…silly, but given the choice I'll go with the apple. The same holds true with cutting up melon or pineapple, but there are alternatives.

Shoprite offers small containers of cut up fruit as do most markets I would imagine. Chunks of cantaloupe, honeydew, pineapple or mixed fruit salads make a nice single serving offering a little variety over buying a whole melon or pineapple and eating nothing but that for the week – not that eating only that is any sort of hardship mind you. The variety is welcome, however, and although the fruit costs quite a bit more when purchased in those little containers, we find the added expense worth it even if it enables my innate laziness. I figure that anything that helps me keep to my healthy path and reduces my dependency on my own will power is welcome.

Although variety is welcome, I have found that the easiest portion for me to control is a single apple cut into sections with an apple corer. Before making my lifestyle change, I had been unaware of the number of different varieties of apples available in the produce section. Granny Smith, Honey Crisp, Red Delicious, Gala, Braeburn, Fuji, oh my goodness the list goes on and on! I'm hard pressed to find an apple I don't like and they're all a perfect portion. Remember the old saying, "an apple a day keeps the doctor away"? I've got to imagine that's a good thing, although I haven't noticed many doctors being kept away.

Chapter Three

B reakfast has been described as the most important meal of the day and I really couldn't afford to be skipping breakfast because of the Januvia. If I allowed my blood sugar levels to fall, I could get dizzy or worse. I was advised to eat whole grains. I had oatmeal every morning while in the hospital. It was tasteless and the consistency of wall paper paste, but if I added raisins and an artificial sweetener I could manage to choke it down.

Before my little incident requiring the cardiologist's attention, my breakfast habits were all over the map. One of my favorite breakfasts was the leftover pizza from the night before cold and right from the box left out on the kitchen counter. Add a tall glass of orange juice and I was set. I really miss pizza; both hot and cold, but I haven't eaten a single slice in over a year. The same is true for a grilled ham and cheese sandwich or toast with peanut butter and let's not forget the classic left over chili! OK, I think it's safe to say that my eating habits weren't much better than the average frat boy at a party school...at least I drank orange juice instead of warm flat beer, but that may have been only marginally better when one considers the calories and fructose contained within.

My wife seems content to begin her day with a bowl of Cheerios and milk, toasted English muffin with jam and a cup of tea each and every morning. I used to love cold cereal but eventually exhibited some difficulty in digesting milk. Once I accepted that I am lactose intolerant, I eschewed milk in my cereal. However I usually ate sugary dry cereal as a snack. Sometimes I would mix it with raisins and munch on it for breakfast. That was not going to be an option any longer. I was determined to eat healthier.

Although my wife rarely alters her morning meal choice, she would understand and accept that I had a desire for variation in my breakfast choices. Still she couldn't understand how I could enjoy my leftovers from the evening meal from the day before until I justified my habits by explaining that I'd learned it to be a common habit of people from many years past. I'd learned that what we commonly recognize as breakfast foods today simply do not go back that far in history. I suspect that I thought that studying the eating habits of my ancestors could justify my eccentric breakfast choices, but I was ready to change all that.

I figured hot cereal each morning was really my best bet for a satisfying breakfast that would stick with me until lunch. Following the formula we'd been taught about subtracting soluble fiber from the carbohydrates and making sure that the resulting number was below 15 grams, my wife and I picked up packets of Kashi Go Lean with seven whole grains as well as their Heart to Heart oatmeal. We tried assortment boxes of instant Irish oatmeal and even the Quaker Oats variety packs. The pre-measured packets aided ease of preparation, which was a good thing since you'll recall that I'm inherently lazy. My wife also seemed to believe that the variety in the hot cereal assortments would assuage my previous desire for leftover pizza, and I admit that I did like the selection.

Early on I might augment the cereal with a Coco multi grain pop cake with a bit of peanut butter if it didn't feel like I'd had enough to eat. I feared falling into the trap of feeling deprived in my efforts to sustain my new eating habits over the long term. I like peanut butter and the Coco multi grain pop cake has a satisfying crunch akin to many snack foods. So along with my hot cereal and pop cake, I would add a tall glass of water, since fruit juice was no longer going to be an option, and I was good to go.

The assortment boxes of hot cereal served me well for months although they seemed sweeter to me than they really needed to be. It took me a while to realize it, but when my wife picked up blueberries, strawberries or bananas, I would cook up some Quaker Oats instant oatmeal and add a little blue packet of Equal along with the fruit de jour. Eventually we stopped buying the Kashi and variety packs altogether and stuck with the large round canister of Quaker Oats instant oatmeal.

I subsequently discovered that I like my oatmeal with a variety of additives. Once when my mother gave us a dried fruit platter, we removed all of the fruit that was sweetened with extra sugar and then I would cut up a few pieces with our kitchen scissors, add Equal and some slivered almonds for a remarkably satisfying breakfast. There was plenty of variety amongst the ingredients I had available to me so I didn't miss the packets of apple cinnamon or maple sugar and I can't help but believe what I'm eating is even healthier. In any event I do find my concoctions filling and satisfying. Oddly enough, I even find the additional effort of preparation inexplicably adds to the whole experience.

Lately in addition to my doctored up oatmeal and a tall glass of water; I might have an individual container of Dannon low fat yogurt (80 calories) or Breakstone's reduced fat cottage cheese (100 calories). Quaker Oats oatmeal has evolved into my habit for breakfast each and every morning for the past year; give or take. Discounting that earlier period during which we tried the Kashi and instant Irish oatmeal, which were both quite tasty, but not any more satisfying that the Quaker Oats once I was through with it.

This had been enough to carry me through until my mid morning snack of the diabetes bar or some grapes. Then the mid morning snacks were eliminated after Dr. Agarwal took me off the Januvia once I had lost enough weight and promised to keep it off; more on that later. Once the midmorning snacks were no longer needed, my breakfast routine was all I required to keep me going until lunch at 12:30.

I got into the routine of scooping a half cup of Quaker Instant Oatmeal into a bowl, adding a cup of water and popping it into the microwave for two minutes. While it cooks, I fill my tall glass with water and take my morning medication and vitamins (Centrum Cardio and fish oil). Six days a week, this is when I prepare my lunch which usually consists of two slices of multi grain bread – all the bread I will allow myself most days – and low sodium cold cuts from the deli such as Boar's Head, or Thuman's ham and turkey, and Alpine Lace Munster cheese. Sometimes I add a slice of tomato, shredded carrots or lettuce if we have some on hand, but often enough my sandwich consists of one slice of turkey, one slice of ham and one slice of cheese if they're sliced medium as is my preference. Thin slices may result in two slices of each of the meats being used; I'm flexible to that extent. Now and then we run out of cold cuts and I need to improvise. Push comes to shove, I will allow myself the occasional peanut butter and jelly sandwich made with Skippy peanut butter and Smucker's sugar free preserves.

After assembly, I place my sandwich in my reusable container and pop it into the refrigerator for later and most mornings I even remember to take it with me when I leave for work. There was a period during which I often forgot my sandwich and had to return for it after visiting the bank. I knew I couldn't chance going without my sandwich, so going back for it was a must. My wife heard about my morning mishaps and came up with a solution that I found quite endearing. She stuck a post-it note to the rear view mirror of my Smart Car that asked "Got Lunch?" I later affixed the note to my sandwich container, which admittedly defeated her intent, but somehow it actually helped me to remember to bring it along with me and gave me a warm and fuzzy feeling as a bonus.

For a while, I also pulled grapes from the stem to put in another matching container; my preference are red seedless, but I wouldn't turn down black or green. Lately I've been eating apples more but this will vary seasonally. I did bring the grapes with me, but I eat the apples only if I get a chance to go home "for lunch". I think that grapes may well be the easiest fruit to eat on the run or between customers at my store. They're self contained and you don't need to worry about them turning color if left unattended for a while. My scheduled time for eating my sandwich has always been 12:30 for the past year. It's the time I decided on when I had to schedule my food intake because of the Januvia and I've adhered to the time ever since.

Since I'm in retail, I'm not always free to take lunch at the same time and there are plenty of times that I might not get to go home for lunch at all. Having lunch with me to eat between waiting on customers was the only way I could assure eating my measured meal at the same time each day. When circumstances do permit a break for lunch, I go home for my apple and perhaps a brief nap. The naps were a must soon after my return to work after my hospital stay; my energy would flag and that half an hour in a comfortable chair helped me make it through the rest of the day and remain upright. These days they're more of a luxury; but a nap is still a welcome respite during a hectic schedule.

In any event, once my oatmeal is done these days; whether I've mixed in a banana, raisins or dried apricots matters little. I then sit down at the table with the book I'm reading at the moment and eat my breakfast; I save the morning paper to read at work. Between the oats, fruit and nuts, there's plenty of fiber in that bowl to keep me feeling full until 12:30 when I'll eat the sandwich I prepared while waiting for my oatmeal to cook and, whether or not I get a chance to go home and eat an apple and take a nap, I'm good until dinner. I have little doubt that becoming a creature of habit was integral to my success.

Sunday is the only day I don't go into work at the store. It is also the only day during which my routine varies most weeks. I still prepare my morning oatmeal for breakfast as I do each and every day for the rest of the week, but I don't prepare a sandwich to take to work because I won't be going to work. Instead, while my oatmeal is in the microwave, I take that time to refill my medication caddy for the week. My expectation is to return home for my 12:30 sandwich most Sundays unless other plans have been made so my routine is maintained.

Chapter Four

A nother ongoing issue for me is salt because of my blood pressure. Although the beta blockers would help to control my pressure, my doctors still advised me to avoid salt. My Doctor also had to admit that totally avoiding salt was nearly impossible. Apparently everything contains salt to one degree or another because it's one of nature's building blocks. Since totally eliminating salt from my diet was not an option, I was admonished that I simply shouldn't add additional salt to anything. In the hospital, I was always given Mrs. Dash to season my food. However, I didn't learn to really appreciate it until I was on my own. Avoiding salt also meant that I couldn't eat most convenience foods. Read those nutrition labels and you'll see than most prepared frozen foods or canned foods are very high in sodium. Even those labeled "heart healthy" contain shocking levels of sodium.

Before my health issues, I frequently ate TV dinners and other microwavable meals for lunch, dinner and sometimes even for breakfast. It was just so much easier to pop something into the microwave than to broil, grill or roast. I work retail hours which usually means that my meals can come at odd hours and I'm often on my own for preparation especially at those odd times. I had to give up the Hot Pockets, frozen lasagna, canned soups, pizza, fried chicken, cheese burgers and fries. However, I didn't have to abandon convenience altogether. I learned to love leftovers reheated in the microwave.

Leftovers can come from a lot of different places. Early on, my wife and I got into the habit of preparing a large meal on Sunday when we were both home together. Perhaps we'd roast a Turkey, bake half a dozen yams (for me, my wife doesn't like yams) and steam a fair amount of broccoli or asparagus. For the rest of the week, I'd place two slices of turkey on a dinner plate along with a yam and some vegetables then pop it in the microwave. Yes, it meant my variety was lacking somewhat, but the food I was now eating was quite a bit better than what I'd been eating when I popped in a Swanson dinner.

Just as easy as roasting a turkey, we could bake or roast a pork loin. We might slice up yams for me and potatoes for her sprinkle them with olive oil and bake them along with the pork loin. We would then add some vegetables and a salad for a lovely meal that left me with plenty of leftovers for the week to be reheated in the microwave as required.

In addition, one pot meals that could also sustain me for a week often include ground turkey. I like to add some kind of beans such as pinto, cannellini or garbanzo (or even a combination of all three), onions, diced salt free tomatoes and whatever else I might have on hand, perhaps carrots or whole wheat pasta. Seasoned liberally with Mrs. Dash extra spicy this makes for a zesty chili-like dish yielding plenty of leftovers for me to microwave.

Another one pot meal might be cut up pieces of chicken with onions, crushed tomatoes and assorted vegetables for something akin to a chicken cacciatore. Scooped onto a plate and heated in the microwave, I could easily eat for the whole week with the results of that one pot. I even discovered that the leftovers often tasted better when reheated a day or two later. I suppose that the flavors are given a better chance to meld as they age. Who knows? In any event, I'm certainly not complaining and I'm eating healthier and very tasty meals.

Besides the sodium issues with prepared foods; I would often over indulge in the quantities. I would think I was being good because I would eat Lean Cuisine or Lean Pockets, but then I would have two because one didn't satisfy me and, what the hell, they had "lean" in the title so that was OK, right? You might recall earlier that I mentioned that I'm an idiot? Consider this to be further confirmation.

And let's not forget the way I would over indulge when we made pasta or a pot of turkey chili. I would stuff myself to the gills with two or even three heaping plates. Sure I felt overstuffed, but I loved every bite as I shoveled it in. I could eat a whole flank steak by myself! The only thing preventing me from doing that was my having to be polite and share with my wife. Is it any wonder that leftovers were a rarity back then?

Often a big dinner like that was followed by a piece of cake or some ice cream and snacking on chips, pretzels or salted nuts in front of the television for the remainder of the evening. Is there any wonder that I had issues with heartburn and acid reflux? We had to purchase Pepcid Complete in the large economy size and I often had to sleep sitting up or be miserable throughout the night.

A large part of my weight loss success was following the doctor's suggestion that I needed to exercise portion control. Instead of eating a second or even a third helping of my ground turkey concoction, I should be satisfied to stop with one. A salad before with a light vinaigrette dressing, instead of the creamy Russian I used to prefer, and some fruit for dessert, instead of ice cream, pudding or cake, certainly helped me to feel full without feeling overly stuffed. Another thing that helped was not eating anything else for the rest of the night. No more snacking in front of the television! By putting a little more distance between my final meal and bed time also meant there was less of a need for the Pepcid Complete…quite the bonus indeed.

Although I had my doubts, Dr. Agarwal, the internist, assured me that I didn't need to be avoiding eating out; I just needed to rethink what I was going to order. Of course, when he asked me for my favorite cuisines he needed to back track a bit. Indian, Thai and Mexican might just prove problematic, but I did learn that I could find something to eat in most restaurants. The trick was to lay off the bread basket, appetizers and desserts. Most of the non-chain restaurants offered some variant of grilled chicken and most are willing to let you double up on the vegetables while avoiding potatoes, pasta or rice. Even when it wasn't on the menu, most restaurants in my area will accommodate my new eating habits and even applaud my restraint.

Another thing that I had to consider was that almost all restaurants in my area tend to serve huge portions as a draw to value conscious patrons. Ordering grilled chicken usually means getting two cutlets. I will often eat half and take the rest home to be popped into the microwave for another meal. A tossed salad to begin the meal is satisfying to me. I was always fond of salad; I just had to make a slight adjustment. I learned to substitute a light vinaigrette dressing for my usual Russian, ranch, Caesar or thousand islands. There's nothing wrong with filling up on salad and it beats out most of the appetizers I might otherwise have ordered. Likewise, there's nothing wrong with filling up on most vegetables as long as they're not swimming in butter or cheese or a deep fried batter, and I find that restaurants don't mind substituting vegetables for potatoes, rice or pasta.

I'm not a total saint when it comes to my diet. I will eat some white rice or a white potato now and then. A white potato baked and dry without butter or sour cream or cheddar cheese or bacon bits or whatever else you might have the habit of filling it with is fine now and then. Roasted potatoes are fine as well, but I lay off of any variation of fried or creamed and I really try to limit mashed. Rice often comes with a dish like a chicken kabob. The chunks of chicken roasted with onions, peppers and tomatoes is really quite healthy and I will allow myself a few forkfuls of the included rice, but will send most of it back to be thrown away no matter how much it rankles to waste food because of my upbringing.

Some restaurants offer a heart healthy option right on the menu, such as sliced turkey, cottage cheese and fruit; or grilled chicken with some leafy greens and a hardboiled egg. Something I've discovered that I like that simply wouldn't have occurred to me a year ago is sliced grilled chicken over a salad. One of my favorites includes salad greens, apple slices, walnuts, white raisins, strawberries and grilled chicken in a raspberry vinaigrette. To me it's like having my salad, dinner and dessert all rolled into one! I now look for that lighter alternative on areas of menus I'd have ignored in the past.

I have noticed more and more restaurants jumping on the healthy diet bandwagon of late. Years ago, during a visit with family in Florida, my wife and I supped in a local Olive Garden. It was a singularly unsatisfying experience at the time and resulted in our avoidance of the chain for the next decade or so. Recently they've begun advertising a section of their menu that features meals that are less than 575 calories. Add to that their all you can eat salad and my wife and I decided to broaden our horizons and give Olive Garden another try. That low calorie section isn't very broad, but it did include a chicken breast in an apricot sauce with sides of broccoli, diced tomatoes and asparagus. It was really quite delightful! I've found that I don't need a huge selection as long as there is something I can eat. We will be going back to the Olive Garden more frequently.

When I have no leftovers and am left on my own for dinner, I will frequently make myself a salad, one broiled chicken breast, or one broiled turkey burger along with a steamer bag of vegetables prepared in the microwave. Check out the nutrition guide on the back. That bag may contain 3 ½ servings, but at 20 to 30 calories a serving, I will often eat that whole bag of green beans! Finishing up with an apple for dessert and I'm content to go back to work for my night on twice a week.

When we eat in without benefit of leftovers to reheat, our dinner might consist of a single boneless pork chop each, a shared baked potato from the microwave; baked beans or corn for her and green beans for me. I usually start with a salad that came prewashed in a bag from Dole. We used to pick these up in Shoprite until we discovered that BJ's offered many times the quantity in a huge tub for about the same price...sometimes the big box stores pay off! To the greens I might add cherry tomatoes, baby carrots, Ocean Spray Craisins, slivered almonds and one of the Ken's light option salad dressings.

I even managed to remain vigilant over the holidays; no easy task, mind you. I was beset by temptation all around me. At Thanksgiving dinner at my sister's house, I managed to limit myself to a green salad augmented by the raw vegetable appetizer that few others seemed to indulge in; two slices of turkey, a yam and broccoli for the main course; and nothing but fruit salad for dessert. I had already lost a considerable amount of weight by then and most of my family and friends understood how much self control I required to have been able to achieve that loss. However, I still heard well meaning suggestions of how it wouldn't kill me to have one little piece of pie, a cookie, one piece of candy or some cheese cake. Such success on my part was deserving of a reward or treat, they told me. Alas, saboteurs are all around you when you are trying to maintain a healthy diet. For me, I know that I can't cheat a little. I don't trust my resolve enough to sample just a taste; I fear pigging out! And I whole heartedly believe that just a little pigging out can undo a whole lot of healthy eating.

Even my subconscious seems worried. Some months back I had a nightmare in which I could not stop myself from eating an entire package of Oreo cookies in a single sitting! I compulsively ate them all even though I wasn't enjoying them. It was as if my body was punishing me for denying it what it craved no matter what I believed was best for me. I awoke in a cold sweat with my heart racing certain I'd undone all the good that I had done over the preceding months. I was relieved it was nothing but a dream and it may actually have reinforced my resolve.

I don't want to gorge on unhealthy foods so the closest I ever came to cheating this past year was both cutlets of my chicken marsala, that few forkfuls of rice pilaf, a baked white potato or an extra helping of fruit salad. Now and then my wife will suggest that I'm deserving of a treat, but when I hear the word "treat" I shudder to think what that might mean. I can't allow myself an indulgence, I must remain vigilant!

Most of my friends and family have been very understanding and supportive of my endeavors. Whenever I was invited for dinner I was usually asked what I could eat so there was always something for me even if everyone else was eating something I wouldn't allow myself. I don't know what I would have done if my host provided nothing but lasagna for dinner. Perhaps I might have made do with salad, assuming a salad was offered, of course. No fruit? No problem, I simply forego dessert and sigh pathetically whilst those around me eat chocolate cake. I made the decision to be good and I'm sticking with it. All my life I'd heard adages suggesting that no one else can do it for me and if I cheat I'd only be hurting myself.

I did come close to that scenario when I was invited to my nephew's eighteenth birthday party. He's studying to be a chef and currently interning in an Italian restaurant. My brother-in-law asked if I'd be able to eat prime rib and I told him that I'd be fine with a small piece since I'm allowed beef once in a while. My nephew showed off his culinary skill by producing a Caesar salad from scratch. I used to love Caesar salad but now fear it too salty for me, so I passed. There was plenty else for me to eat. I filled up on the vegetables others didn't seem to want. I never feel guilty about finishing off the vegetables before they're sent back to the kitchen. After the main course they gave me an apple for dessert while everyone else had cookies and cake.

My wife and I have gotten around the problem of beef by planning ahead. We used to eat a lot of flank steak. The two of us could polish off a good size flank steak with me eating the bulk of it as I mentioned earlier. I won't do that anymore, but that would still leave the problem of leftovers which I shouldn't be eating in subsequent days so soon after eating the original meal. It just took a little planning to come up with a workable solution. What we do now is to cut the flank steak into four equal pieces to freeze individually for four separate meals with no leftovers. Problem solved!

I don't want to offend a host and I know that I can get evangelical about my healthy diet to an obnoxious degree, but I also know that I have to be extreme in my vigilance because halfway measures simply will not suffice for me. I don't believe that I can fall off the wagon and then get right back on. OK, maybe I can, but why chance it? I think it better that I do everything I can to stay aboard the wagon in the first place. If that makes it intolerable to be around me, so be it. I have to do what works for me and I think that my success justifies my obsessive self control. Fortunately, my family and friends appear understanding and haven't stopped inviting me for dinner yet...

Chapter Five

O f course, my eating habits weren't the only thing that required modification. There were other parts of the equation that needed to be adjusted. I hadn't climbed on a scale in years and would have had no idea how much I weighed when this all began had I not gotten weighed in the hospital. I imagine that it's not all that unusual for those of us who are obese to avoid weighing ourselves. It's so much easier to ignore our weight if we don't know how much we weigh. I certainly appeared to follow that belief. Even after I began to modify my eating habits, I avoided weighing myself at first. Sure, I couldn't help but notice that my clothes were fitting looser. Those around me commented that I appeared to be losing some girth. Even my doctors noticed my weight loss and commented on it as I cinched my belt tighter to hold up my baggy jeans.

My wife and I were already keeping a journal in which we recorded my sugar level, blood pressure and pulse. Dr. Agarwal, the internist, suggested that I begin recording my weight as well. He understood my reluctance to get on a scale and didn't want me to weigh myself compulsively, but thought twice a week would be a good guideline. So two weeks after leaving the hospital, I climbed on the scale at home for the first time in years and recorded my weight at 242 pounds. I'd lost eighteen pounds in pretty short order. Soon after that, my wife dug out all of the jeans she'd been storing in our shed out back as I'd outgrown them on the way up. Now I was trying on progressively smaller sizes as I began to reverse the trend. I found I liked the feeling of clothing that was too loose on me after suffering those that were too tight for so long. However, even as I shrank, I was reluctant to adopt tighter clothes. It often took those around me to keep pointing out to me that my clothes were looking baggy and it was time for a smaller size for me to make the changes.

Dr. Agarwal, the internist, also suggested that I needed to begin to exercise. He cautioned that I still had to take it easy following my cardiac episode and he didn't want me to over exert myself. He liked that I had a strider machine left over from all those years before called the Gazelle. Upon that machine, I could swing my arms and legs for a workout as strenuous as I chose to make it. We decided to keep it low impact for five minutes two to three times a week in the beginning and gradually increase it as I felt able.

As I mentioned before, I still tired easily and needed to take naps even after I returned to work some weeks later. I kept up doing the Gazelle and I was making healthy changes to my diet. I was still formulating a sustainable pattern of eating and exercise. I knew it wouldn't do me any good unless I could come up with something I could maintain long term and I'd proven before that the long term habit was where I needed the most work. I did hold out hope for exercising at home rather than relying on trips to the gym which I knew from past experience might not last.

Being able to fit into successively smaller jeans was positive reinforcement. Seeing results encouraged me to persevere with my sensible eating and exercise. As the weather began to warm, I came up with alternatives to the Gazelle. The first thing I did after my cardiologist allowed me to return to driving, and just before I was to return to work, was to drive over to Van Saun Park to take a walk around the duck pond. It was a bit of a struggle, but I made one complete circuit which was six tenths of a mile according to a sign posted along the path.

I've always liked walking and now that I'd had my angioplasty it looked as though I'd be able to do more of it without suffering ill consequences. At least I wasn't gasping for breath after my circuit around the pond. My legs hurt a little, but not as much as before my hospital stay. A little cramping, but thankfully the sciatica from before seemed to be eased. Still, after returning to work I would have a lot less free time for that sort of thing so I needed to get creative.

My wife frequently drives when we go out; she just prefers to be behind the wheel rather than riding as a passenger most times when we go somewhere. The weather was pleasant enough, so I began having her drop me off a half a mile from home forcing me to walk the rest of the way. When we ate in, I began taking walks around my neighborhood following dinner. Sometimes my wife would join me to further encourage the habit. I began going grocery shopping with my wife on Sunday and I would push the cart just to keep moving. Eventually we began visiting parks on Sundays for a walk around the pond following the grocery shopping. There are several parks in our area and I believe we've visited them all at least once now. Each has something else to offer it, but variety is what they offer most of all to keep boredom at bay.

My walks gradually became more frequent and of longer duration. Since most parks won't let you walk in them after dark, I find my walks in the evening involve wandering my neighborhood. I take different routes exploring as I go and I've become ubiquitous enough that neighbors even blocks away have begun waving to me as I pass. Occasionally a different route will mean that I lose my way temporarily, but since that leads to a longer walk as I find my way again I think it a good thing. Now and then my wife will grow concerned when my walks are of longer duration than she'd anticipated, but she's gotten used to my disappearances and has been witness to the positive results.

These days, weather permitting, my wife now leaves me off a mile to a mile and a half from home. However, when the weather becomes inclement once more, I'll retreat to the Gazelle. Lately, I've been trying to exercise every day whether it's a walk in the park, neighborhood, or fifteen minutes to a half hour on the Gazelle. I've also added calisthenics, dumbbells and resistance exercises. Often when I walk in the park now, I'll stop between laps to do a set of push-ups on one of the benches. I've even found that I can exercise at work when things are slow. I can do pushups, walk the aisles and climb the stairs. I find the more I do the easier it is to do it. Some would call that physical conditioning, I'd imagine.

I'm prepared to face the fact that I'm no athlete and I'll probably forego being the worst softball player in the league this time around, but I can't help but be pleased that my continuing exercise and healthy diet is lending itself to an improved sense of well being. When I'm alone in my walk through the park or around the neighborhood, it gives me the opportunity to ponder life's many mysteries. It's almost like meditation for me…

Chapter Six

As I fell into my routines of healthy eating, plenty of rest and moderate exercise I gradually began to note some ancillary benefits. I was losing weight at a rate of a pound or two a week, but more interesting were the reduction of swelling in my hands and the disappearance of my sciatica. For years I'd heard the complaint of every overweight individual who visited their doctor. No matter what was wrong with you, it could easily be alleviated with the loss of a bit of weight. I recently saw a Hagar the Horrible comic strip in which Doctor Zook recommended weight loss to solve Hagar's dandruff. Silly, perhaps, but I was seeing results from my weight loss beyond my clothes fitting looser. Among other things, the weight loss has appeared to alleviate my sleep apnea. At least I'm told that I no longer snore like a woodsman's chain saw. And silly though it may seem it feels as though the cab of my Smart Car has gotten roomier.

Between the weight loss and the meds I was taking, there was also a noticeable alteration of my internal thermostat. I felt chilled at any temperature below seventy-seven degrees. The winter months saw me dressing in multiple layers against the cold, but when summer came around I found myself more tolerant of the extreme heat than anyone else around me. At times I wondered if that was to be my new super power.

People all around me began noticing that there was less of me to love. By the middle of May I was down to 220 pounds, forty pounds off my high in about four months and about six inches off my waist. I was frequently hearing some variation of "Wow, you've lost a lot of weight, how'd you do it?" Of course I quickly learned that no one really wanted to hear the details of how I did it. Most were hoping for a magic pill or were looking for an opening to tell me that they'd lost ten pounds recently and were trying to lose ten more, yadda, yadda, yadda… At first I would go into detail about my new habits until their eyes began to glaze over with obvious boredom. Gradually I got into the habit of replying that it was due to careful diet and exercise unless I'm pressed for more details.

People were telling me that I looked good with increasing frequency which began to inspire my sarcastic side. I started channeling Billy Crystal as Fernando from Saturday Night Live. Affecting a cheesy accent I would declare that it is more important to look good than to feel good…and I look marvelous! That was usually good for a few chuckles, but it became prophetic as my dizzy episodes increased and I began getting some mild chest pains when I exerted myself; nothing like before, but still a matter of some concern.

On my next visit to Dr. Agarwal, the internist, I was standing in his examining room when he came in and told me that I looked fantastic and asked how I did it. I told him that I just did what he'd suggested and he responded "No really, how'd you do it?" I finally convinced him that I'd just been following his advice by reducing my intake of salt, eliminating sugar, controlling my portions and exercising a bit. He marveled over my success. He insisted that no one ever listened to anything he suggested. He also listened to my list of physical complaints.

"Well, you called my bluff," Dr. Agarwal began, "I'm going to have to take you off the Januvia. However if you put any of the weight back on or your sugar spikes; you're going right back on it!" He then admitted that he tells all his patients that he can take them off some of their medications if they adjust their eating habits and lose some weight, but usually they fail to do so and he doesn't have to follow through. Apparently I'm his only patient that ever did what he recommended, or so he claimed. Also because of my weight reduction, he had to lower the dosages of the Metoprolol tartr since the dosage is based on weight. It was hoped that these changes would help with the dizziness and chest pain, although he suggested some pain might be expected in view of my procedures from a couple of months before. My body might still be adjusting to the stents. This was also the first time that Dr. Agarwal would suggest that I should write a book about my weight loss and he would make it required reading for all of his patients.

Being off the Januvia meant I no longer had to concern myself with a mid morning snack and I did get relief from much of the dizziness. My wife continued testing my sugar and I've maintained acceptable levels ever since. However, the chest pains persisted even though I tried to ignore them. My wife insists that I have always had a high tolerance for pain that will ultimately be my undoing. Others have suggested that it's a male pattern of idiocy and the avoidance of inconvenient medical intervention. Inevitably, the chest pains would prove to be a problem that could no longer be ignored.

Sometime in June, I had a particularly intense episode that had me reaching for the Nitroglycerin. The following morning, I phoned Dr. Agarwal's service and left a message about my chest pain from the night before. He called right back and insisted that I check into the ER and get it tested assuring me that it was probably nothing of concern and I'd be home by late afternoon. It was nothing but a precaution; my wife and I even made plans to go out for dinner and a movie after the test.

He had me request a specific test for a particular enzyme. After the test, the young doctor in the ER told me that I wasn't going anywhere and immediately admitted me. I had visits that day from both Dr. Agarwal's, neither of whom was mincing words; the enzyme they'd tested for indicated that I'd had a heart attack. Both assured me that I'd been an exemplary patient and that this was a freak occurrence…I think that they were worried I'd take this set back as an excuse to return to my evil ways since being good was apparently no guarantee of success.

I had another heart attack on the operating table while Dr. Agarwal's cardiac team went to work on me. Another clot was found and cleared and yet another stent was put in place. The cardiologist told me that I shouldn't have accepted any chest pain and hoped that I would continue to lose weight, eat right and exercise.

Whether this was a new clot that had formed above a previously placed stent or a clot that had simply been missed some months before is open to debate to this very day. I do know that I've been relatively pain free since the last procedure and I accepted it as only a temporary setback. There was little or no permanent damage to my heart and my recovery time proved much quicker than the time before. Perhaps the weight loss, from healthy nutrition and exercise, along with a faithful regimen of medication had paid dividends. I accepted it as such and continued doing what I had been doing without very much of a gap.

I was even more determined to continue with my healthier diet and went right back to regular exercise after a brief convalescence. I made up my mind not to back slide. My problems were of my own making and all of my doctors were doing all they could to keep me on the road to recovery. This was no excuse to return to my far worse habits of a half a year before.

Chapter Seven

At the time of my relapse, I had lost over fifty pounds and by the end of July I entered what my sister referred to as my "one-derfuls". From that point forward, the first number of my weight would be a one. I was determined that the first number would never be a two again, there was no looking back. I was sticking to my new eating habits and I was intending to step up the exercising adding more for my upper body to my walking and time on the Gazelle.

Soon after the first number of my weight became a one, the first number of the waist on my jeans became a three! I was reluctant to begin wearing the next size smaller each time because I still remembered struggling to fit into ever larger sizes. It wasn't until people were commenting about how loosely my jeans were hanging upon me that I would even consider the next size smaller, consequently my clothes fit loosely even when I opted for a smaller size which probably led to many people commenting that I was losing weight at a prodigious pace.

Although my wife had retained my smaller sized jeans and stored them away, that hadn't been the case with shirts. She seemed to be having fun selecting a whole new wardrobe of shirts for me to wear with my jeans. Pretty early on, the size 2X shirts in my closet were feeling pretty loose followed by any 1X. We were intrigued to learn that 1X is very often somewhat larger than XL, but both gave way to large before the fall. I'm now wearing medium sized shirts. The changing weather dictated some of her choices naturally enough and it's fortunate that I usually dress quite casually so there was little need for more expensive attire. However, when the warmer weather rolls around I have to wonder if the large short sleeve knits from last year are still going to fit or if there will be a new round of acquisitions.

While my wife had saved my jeans; I held onto more eccentric wardrobe items. As the weather grew chillier I was able to fish out a leather flight jacket someone had picked up for me at the Air Force PX. One of my favorite coats is a 1950s era army surplus heavy wool great coat from the Belgian army that I obtained several years ago for the princely sum of $15! I hadn't been able to fit into it for at least a half a dozen years and was delighted to begin wearing it again as winter weather rolled around. That coat attracts a lot of positive attention from everyone around me and was one of my favorite ancillary benefits of losing so much weight. The coat practically screams military, so I added a dragon and a mermaid pin to the lapels. It still speaks to people who are often telling me that the coat reminds me of one worn by their ancestor in mother Russia or Afghanistan, or fill in the blank. Apparently no one checks the buttons which may well be the only difference from one army coat to another; mine has the rampant lions of the Belgian infantry.

I recently decided that I might need a suit soon. I don't dress up very much; a flannel shirt and a pair of jeans serve me well enough at work and we rarely go anywhere that requires a jacket and tie. However, one can't really dress that way at a formal affair such as a wedding or, heaven forbid, a funeral. The last suit I purchased was for my nephew's wedding almost a year and a half before. It was actually two suits purchased at The Men's Warehouse during one of their frequent buy one get one free sales. I actually never got the chance to wear the other of the two, or most of the shirts I selected to go with them. My closet was getting a little overly full, so I decided to donate most of the suits and jackets I had in smaller sizes. The exceptions were specialty suits I'd purchased to wear as costumes. Unfortunately, I don't feel comfortable wearing a fire engine red zoot suit or cut away tails to your average wedding or funeral.

So I recently went out and bought a new suit at the Jos. A Banks outlet store nearby us in The Bergen Town Center outlet mall. It fit me beautifully right off of the rack and it was a 42 short! Those last two suits I purchased before my nephew's wedding were both 50 portly short. The jacket practically fit around both me and my wife together when I tried them on before heading out to buy my new suit. At least the ties I purchased back then still fit, but that's about all. Along with ninety-five pounds, I've lost about fourteen inches off of my waist and eight inches off of my chest. I now even have dimples when I smile.

As my weight declined, I kept trimming back my beard. With my face getting thinner as well as the rest of my body, I began to think that the thick, bushy beard of my Santa Claus look was overpowering. The last time I sported a full beard, albeit trimmer, my weight had slipped below 190 pounds. I now sport a goatee, but I arrived there in stages and gradually trimmed it shorter and shorter. I began posting before and after pictures of my progress on Facebook; the first was just before I went goatee. Each time I did so, the response was greater than the time before which naturally encouraged me even further. Everyone roots for a loser as long its weight they're losing, or so it seems to me now.

I was already below 200 pounds the first time I discussed a goal weight with Dr. Agarwal who once again suggested that I needed to write a book. I thought 170 was achievable but he worried that might be too extreme. Initially he suggested 180 and then thought 175 might be an acceptable compromise.

While at work during a slow period, my cousin and I visited a website that featured a chart about BMI or body mass index. According to that chart, I should weigh in around 155 at my 5'7" height and now, at the first anniversary of my original hospital stay of 2012, I'm flirting with 165 pounds. The 175 Dr. Agarwal had suggested was admittedly an arbitrary figure although he does believe the weight charts are not always realistic.

On my last check up, Dr. Agarwal accepted my weight now being below his suggested goal as a good thing. Adding to that was a blood test that revealed textbook perfect numbers across the board and the good doctor wanted to know how much more I intended to lose, so I told him about the BMI and discussions I'd had with my sister about my weight loss intentions.

My sister has asked me this question on more than one occasion. She wanted to know if I planned to eat differently if I achieved any particular goal. I assured her that, since I don't really consider myself to be on a "diet", I have no plan to change my new eating habits. I eat the way I do because I believe it to be in my best interest for continued good health. Pleased with my response she suggested that my body will dictate my eventual weight. Sooner or later, I will stop losing weight once my body adjusts to the calories I consume and the exercise with which I burn those calories. I will find a weight level naturally. I'm still sort of hoping to get down to at least 160 because I like the thought of having lost 100 pounds; it's such a nice round number after all.

At this point, I'm still getting a lot of comments that involve the "Wow you've lost a lot of weight" and "How did you do it?" variety, but many are more interesting. One young mother was visiting my store with her little one in tow. She was effusive in her praise of my achievement and asked her young son if he was impressed with my weight loss. He wouldn't look at me. He kept looking down at his feet and finally remarked in a sorrowful little voice, "He doesn't look like Santa anymore." Apparently I'd lost some of the magic along with the weight, at least in his estimation.

Another long time customer kept looking at me from different locations within the store. When she finally came forward to pay for her purchases she asked me if the store was under new ownership. I assured her that it was not. Then she asked if I was related to the fat guy with the big beard that used to work there. When I told her that I was the same guy, she could hardly believe it and then the conversation followed the "Wow, you've lost a lot of weight." And "How did you do it?" formula.

I usually leave a copy of Santa 17 on the front counter in hopes of attracting the attention of potential buyers. There's a photograph of me on the back cover and I've been using it lately to remind people of what I looked like more than a year before. That woman who couldn't believe that I was the same guy was fascinated by my picture on the back of my book as a visual aid. So much so, in fact, that she purchased a copy of the book. Who knew that weight loss could be such an effective marketing strategy?

Someone who had bought a copy of Santa 17 about a year ago recently asked me if I was any relation to the author of the book. I told her that I was intimately related. In fact, I am that self same author! She too was amazed by my weight loss and I was delighted that she had enjoyed reading my book, a win win!

My cousin has told me that several of our long time customers are afraid to ask me about my weight loss. A number of them feared that my weight loss was due to one wasting illness or another and simply couldn't face a depressing conversation. After he assures them that the change was intentional, they're eager to learn how I did it, hoping of course that it was some magic pill that required no sacrifice of any sort. I do hate to burst their bubble by declaring the result is due to careful diet and exercise, but I've always been willing to go into detail with anyone who demonstrates genuine interest.

A number of people have suggested that I look too skinny, that I've already lost too much or I can't possibly believe that I need to lose anymore. I understand that I look quite a bit different. I'm occasionally surprised when I see my reflection in a mirror. How can others recognize me when I don't always recognize myself? I still expect to see the fatter me and I'm still getting used to being smaller. I'm often surprised at the smaller spaces I can fit into such as the narrower aisles in my store. Sometimes when I pick up a pair of jeans I fear that they will be too small for me to get into until I slip them on and realize I could take the next size smaller.

Chapter Eight

G radually the pace of my weight loss slowed as we had all imagined it would, but I was still losing inches as exercise continued to tone my body. By March of 2013 I was wearing 34" waist jeans and they were not snug.

As spring rolled around again, my wife and I realized that the short sleeve shirts from the year before were now going to be far too large. A size large fit me fine then, but the long sleeve shirts of winter had been mediums and now they were fitting loosely enough that we wondered if I may now require a size small. Having to buy new clothing is probably the greatest cost of weight loss success.

Beware the "ides of April" doesn't have the same ring to it as the famous line from the Shakespeare play about Julius Caesar. It is plenty ominous, however, because so many think of it as "tax day" since it is the day by which most of us mere mortals are required to have had our taxes filed. For me, however, April 15, 2013 was the first day I recorded a weight below 160 pounds! I had lost 100 pounds, that arbitrary yet magical number I had hoped to achieve.

The Sunday before April 15th, my wife and I went for a long walk in Van Saun Park. When we returned home, I did some calisthenics and threw around the dumbbells for a bit, I even did fifteen minutes on the gazelle. Dinner for me was a full serving of steamed chicken and string beans with a bit of brown rice that we brought in from a Chinese restaurant. I finished with a Granny Smith apple for dessert.

I needed to mail a couple of letters on April 15th. After navigating through the long lines of tax payers at the post office on that morning, I headed to the bank. My weight loss is often a topic of discussion amongst the tellers at the bank I frequent and that morning was no different. I welcomed the usual questions and comments since I had the news of my 160 pound weigh in. Another fellow visiting a different teller was telling her that he would be bringing them some cannoli soon. After he left, I learned that he was their new favorite customer since he kept bringing in boxes of bakery treats that he acquired at the bakeries he visited in his capacity as a health inspector.

Last week it had been éclairs and my teller admitted she'd eaten five of them! What amused me most about this was how they often complain how difficult it is for them to lose weight and how much easier it is for me because I'm a man and men lose weight so much easier than women. I mention that I haven't eaten a single éclair or cannolo in over a year, but I don't think they made the connection.

One day, when my sister was in the store with me, a customer came in that recognized my car out front but couldn't connect me to the image she of me in her mind. She asked where the owner of the Smart Car with the Looney Tunes characters and wind-up key was to be found. After I told her that I was indeed that self same individual, she informed me that I've lost a lot of weight and asked me how I did it...you know the routine by now. A new twist was added when my sister entered the discussion telling all around us that "He eats like a bird! Ask him when the last time was that he had a piece of cake..."

Another woman in line remarked "He couldn't eat like a bird, birds eat constantly!" suggesting that birds must consume more than their own weight during the course of a day and that would obviously be no way for someone to lose a hundred pounds.

June of 2013 marked the anniversary of my last cardiac episode and I was informed that I needed to go in for a Nuclear Stress test and echocardiogram as the standard follow up. As a nurse shaved my chest so that the electrodes could be affixed, she asked if I exercise. I told her that I did so every day now. She remarked that she could tell...a little positive reinforcement, to be sure. The technician who injected the dye suggested that I might need to eat something to get it to circulate, but I refused the graham crackers or oatmeal cookies she offered opting for the grapes I'd brought with me instead. A second round of dye administered an hour later brought the suggestion that I needed to eat something again, but I had no more grapes. She couldn't believe that I wasn't hungry and remarked that it was probably the reason that I was so "skinny"...more positive reinforcement.

So, following her suggestion, I wandered downstairs to the lobby café wearing my clinical hospital robe with the understanding that they're used to seeing patients in search of sustenance. The café looks as much like a news stand as anything else. He had lots of snacks like chips, cookies and candy. There were assorted premade sandwiches and, surprisingly, a bowl of fruit. I asked if any of the sandwiches were on whole grain bread and he offered me two options from the back; tuna or turkey and Swiss cheese. My turkey and cheese sandwich was labeled as made with Boars head deli products and included lettuce and one thin slice of tomato. There were condiments, which I discarded, in packets below the sandwich. The vendor indicated a price of $6.00 which included a bag of chips or a piece of fruit; apples, oranges and bananas making up the selection. My sandwich was surprisingly tasty and the banana a satisfying extra. Not only did this reinforce the notion that I could eat almost anywhere, but the dye circulated perfectly with no more impediment to the test.

It has been over a year and a half since I made the decision to change my habits in a positive way and I'm finding it easier and easier to stick with it. However, I realize that I must remain vigilant. Complacency could prove to be my enemy. Better than avoiding temptation is to find that I'm no longer tempted at all and that was actually the case with the cookies and crackers I had been offered in the cardiac testing lab.

Because of scheduling issues, I had now seen three different cardiologists from Dr. Agarwal's group. For the follow up to my stress test I was finally to see Dr. Agarwal again for the first time in the year since he performed my last angioplasty. He had no idea who I was. He asked why I was there and I related my saga brining him up to date. He was amazed and had his assistant run an EKG. I was told I'd aced my stress test – apparently all my studying had paid off – and he was pleased with what he'd seen on my EKG. I was told to stop taking Effient and Amlodipine immediately and there's some indication that other meds will follow in their wake after the results of a blood test.

At a party to celebrate my nephew's graduation from high school, I was briefly surrounded by friends and in-laws of my sister, who hadn't seen me since the last party over a year before, and were marveling over my apparent transformation. "105 pounds?! You've lost an entire person!" proclaimed one of my sister's brothers-in-law. To put things in perspective, his wife chimed in that she weighed 105 pounds suggesting, I suppose, that she might be the person I'd lost.

So that's my story; the secret to my success. I believe that if I stick to my new habits of healthy diet and exercise I will continue to benefit in myriad ways. If Dr. Agarwal, the internist, is correct, many of my fellow baby boomers who have likewise fallen victim to heart disease might also improve their health by eating a healthier diet and getting into the habit of regular exercise. If reading this book inspires a few to find their own path to a healthier lifestyle it will have been worth my effort in writing down my experiences.

Michael Grapin
P.O. Box 194
Paramus, NJ 07653-0194
MAGrapin@optonline.net